Tai Chi Techniques for

Correcting Your Posture While Sitting, Standing, and Lying Down

by Dr. Money

FREE YOUR MIND AND BODY

"Having dealt with both Scoliosis and Kyphosis as a teen—to the point of wearing a hip-to-chin back brace for several years—by the time I hit college, I suffered from chronic back pain. Though I was not yet 22 years old, some mornings my back hurt so much I couldn't get out of bed. The doctors told me I'd have to learn to live with chronic back pain, because my spine couldn't be fixed. Not a happy prospect at such a young age.

Then I discovered Tai Chi. It literally changed my life. Within a few weeks of learning how to align and relax my spine, the pain lessened. After a few months of diligent practice, I was pain-free for the first time in ten years. Now, in my mid-forties, I still credit what I learned from Tai Chi with giving me a life I might not have had."

-Jeffe Kennedy, International author and Neurophysiologist

When I was 30 years old I worked as a research scientist and spent many hours every day looking through a microscope. As a result of this tedious work I began to suffer from spinal compression which caused my neck to become stiff and painful. I also frequently experienced dizziness and nausea. The older researchers told me this was a very common work-related injury with microbiologists and advised me to go see a chiropractor. After several treatments my neck was looser, but I continued to experience neck and lower back pain due to my poor posture. After a month of doing Quiet Standing following the Tai Chi alignment principles I realized an enormous release of tension from my body that left me feeling 10 years younger. I want to tell the whole world about it!

-David Money, Doctor of Oriental Medicine

Catalina Acupuncture Press
7 Avenida Vista Grande B-7
PMB #457
Santa Fe, NM 87508
505-288-1711
www.catalinaacupuncture.com

Disclaimer: The exercises in this book are not intended to be used to as a substitute for medical treatment. Anyone who engages in these exercises does so at their own risk. Prior to undertaking any physical exercise program, we advise you to consult your physician.

DEDICATION

To the most influential person I've ever known—my love
and partner in crime, Jeffe Kennedy, who extended her passion,
wisdom, and persistence in driving me toward my goals.

CONTENTS

When the sacrum is straight
the body is agile
and the spirit ascends
Tai Chi Classics

ACKNOWLEDGMENTS

Special thanks to all my teachers who so generously shared the mastery of their art. They were all truly experts of their craft.

And my sincere gratitude to all the students I've had the privilege to train—and learn from—over the years.

INTRODUCTION

Back and neck pain—who *doesn't* suffer from them from time to time? Current statistics reveal that fully 80% of the U.S. population will experience some sort of back problem during their lives. Unfortunately, with our fast paced, high-tech, never-slow-down society, we've adopted the attitude that it's normal—even natural!—to have aches and pains by the time we're 40!

What's even worse is that some doctors are now telling people there's nothing they can do about their pain this side of surgery.

Who wants to feel old and decrepit at 40?

Do not—I repeat in capital letters—DO NOT buy into the static that your body is worn out and irreparably broken!

There is **zero** evidence that your body should fall apart at age 40—*or* at age 60 or 70. Here are just a few noteworthy examples of people who have accomplished tremendous physical feats at 60 years of age and beyond:

Jack LaLanne swam across Long Beach Harbor *while towing 70 row boats with passengers* at age 70.

Roger Brockenbrough, age 77, has entered and completed 200+ triathlons—and continues to enter them!

And Barry Finlay climbed Mount Kilimanjaro on his 60th birthday.

These are just three examples out of countless 60+ year old high achievers who have proven that the human body continues to be strong and resilient as it ages.

What do super achievers have that most other people lack? *The right attitude!* They embrace the notion that their body is robust and built to last.

Since you're reading this book, it's a fair guess you're concerned about the quality of your future. You may have tried every procedure known to conventional medicine to reduce your neck or back pain with little to no success. If your intuition is telling you there must be another way to get rid of your pain and restore your sense of vigorous wellbeing, there is! Best of all, it's drug free. It's called Tai Chi.

Why I tackled writing a book about pain and Tai Chi

I feel fortunate to have learned potent natural methods of healing from some stellar Tai Chi practitioners. And I believe you should have access to the same knowledge because what I've learned can help you improve your comfort level and restore your physical and mental well being. (With the current cost of health care, you need every advantage you can get!)

I want you to feel good again. Because when you feel good, you inspire others to feel good. So if the information I share here helps a hundred people feel good, those 100 people will help a thousand people feel good—all from helping them improve their posture!

So let's talk about posture.

Posture

For starters, what is posture? The Oxford Universal English Dictionary defines posture as "a relative disposition of parts, the position and carriage of the body and limbs, a state of being, or a mental or spiritual attitude."

In other words, your state of mind has a major effect over your posture.

Like your muscles, your body has been trained to a particular pattern, one that is now causing you considerable pain. Left unattended, especially after an injury or if you continually perform a physical task in an odd position, the harder it will be to change your posture *unless you have a proven set of ideas worthy of embracing*. Remember: better posture will come into being from the ideas your mind happily embraces!

There is an ancient set of highly effective ideas for improving posture that comes from generations of Tai Chi masters. The ancient alignment principles of Tai Chi provide a step by step 'how to' guide for building a posture that is strong and resilient. This system has been formulated, tested, and proven by Tai Chi masters over thousands of years.

In the past 50 years Tai Chi has become a highly respected martial art in the US. In China it has gained fame as "The Grand Ultimate" because the discipline is believed to contain both the *yin* and the *yang* of a robust lifestyle. Traditionally *yin* and *yang* represent balanced relationships: hot and cold, movement and stillness, tension and relaxation, the elements we can observe in nature and within our own bodies. It is believed that the study of Tai Chi gives us control over all *yin* and *yang* qualities. More than 121 different styles of Tai Chi have been identified and taught in China across the millennia.

In the U.S. Tai Chi is depicted as a series of slow, gentle physical movements and described by many authors as a form of moving meditation. As with any philosophical system, there is debate among scholars about the exact origin of the art, but for the purposes of this book, we can ignore the static. (But for those of you interested in the history of Tai Chi, I'll provide excellent references in the appendix.)

Tai Chi is appropriate for people of all ages. Although typically practiced in a standing position, the principles can also be practiced while sitting or lying down.

What distinguishes Tai Chi from other martial arts

The distinguishing characteristic of Tai Chi is its focus on building a supple body and mind. Many people mistakenly think the benefits of Tai Chi come from the graceful movements they see. Although important, the movements themselves tend to distract people from the wonderful principles of good posture which is the foundation of all Tai Chi practice. Free graceful movements aren't the goal; they're the outward effect of the release of tension from mind and body.

In this guide, I'll walk you through the ideas and exercises that foster a strong, resilient, and supple Tai Chi posture. You'll learn the essential ideas of alignment and how to practice them. You'll gain an understanding of the Chinese idea of *sung*, "to be strong as a mountain". I'll discuss the sympathetic and parasympathetic nervous system and why it's important to your posture and health. I'll talk about what to expect from your practice and how to apply a breathing technique to release your lower back tension. I'll finish by covering how often you should practice and give you some ideas to boost your strength and energy.

CHAPTER 1
THE NERVOUS SYSTEM

The human nervous system is an astounding mechanism that functions as a high-speed communication system. Made of thousands of delicate fibers, it can be easily damaged by injury, disease, inadequate nutrition, drugs, and lazy posture.

The central portion of the nervous system controls physical movement and is under conscious control. The peripheral nervous system (also known as the autonomic system) regulates the organs and glands and is under subconscious control. Because of the autonomic portion, we don't have to consciously regulate our heart beat; Mother Nature does that.

The peripheral nervous system is also divided into *sympathetic* and *parasympathetic* systems which work harmoniously (like *yin* and *yang*) to balance each other.

The system of Tai Chi I'll present here focuses on structural components that are essential to activating the healing system of your body (your parasympathetic nervous system). By correctly aligning your body with these ancient principles, you can unblock your nervous system and allow it to function properly.

"Few people understand the importance of the nervous system to overall health. Fewer still know how to align their bodies to receive maximum function from them."

CHAPTER 2
BENEFITS OF TAI CHI

In his book *Cheng Tzu's Thirteen Treatises on Tai Chi chuan*, professor Cheng Man Ching listed the following benefits:

- Increased blood circulation

- Increased energy

- Takes pressure off spinal nerves and joints

- Activates sympathetic nervous system

- Slows the heart rate

Other notable Tai Chi teachers have stated that Tai Chi practice also:

- Raises the spirit

- Improves peace of mind

- Increases body weight in thin people

- Decreases weight in overweight people

- Clears the mind and improves thinking

- Promotes digestion

- Softens the blood vessels

- Cleans the digestive organs

- Promotes nutritional assimilation

- Mends bones and marrow

- Strengthens the skin

CHAPTER 3
PRACTICE TIPS

In ancient China, Tai Chi was considered a gentlemen's art. This statement underscores an important concept and offers a clue about how to practice Tai Chi.

A "gentleman" was defined as a person of high class who used his mind (instead of brute force) to accomplish tasks. The gentleman concept informs us as to how to practice Tai Chi: *apply finesse rather than force*. A gentleman exhibited finesse in thought and action, giving the impression that he was never overly concerned about danger. He was relaxed and aware of what was going on around him at all times. His movements appeared graceful and elegant.

One of the most important Tai Chi manuals, *The Tao Te Ching*, speaks of awareness as the quality of being "watchful like men crossing a winter stream". This statement indicates that Tai Chi practice should be approached with a *heightened state of mental awareness*. By practicing in this way, you'll quicken your sensory perception which will lead to finessing your actions.

Finesse is a crucial quality in Tai Chi training. *Finesse means to do things in an artful or refined way.*

To get an idea of what finesse is, watch a cat play with a mouse or a snake. Cats have refined movements; if you study them you'll notice the crisp, swift precision of their actions.

Finesse requires precise action without hesitation. Finesse develops from paying close attention to detail and correct practice. For example, when you sharpen a knife blade, you must carefully and gradually take off layers until the blade is perfectly beveled to a sharpened edge. A dull knife makes a butcher's job difficult; its jagged edge creates resistance as it cuts and tears. A properly-sharpened knife encounters little resistance and adds the appearance of artfulness and grace to the butcher's movements. In the same way, building a strong, supple posture requires that we be artful in our approach, training mind and body rather than forcing things to happen.

CHAPTER 4
RELAXATION

One of the most important aspects of Tai Chi practice is allowing your body to become relaxed. But you can't **make** yourself relax—your mind will resist a direct command to do so. Emile Coue, the famous French hypnotherapist said, "When the imagination and the will are in opposition, the imagination always wins the day."

Relaxation happens automatically when your body is properly aligned. Repetition, not force, is the key to releasing the tension in your body. Repetition sends you a powerful message, telling your mind and body that *its new pattern is relaxation.* To this end, *always undertake the exercises from the attitude that* **you're allowing your body to relax.** If you practice this way, you'll quickly notice changes in your body, attitude and sense of wellbeing.

You can encourage the attitude of relaxation by finding a quiet place, preferably first thing in the morning, and either standing or sitting there. Allow your arms to hang by your sides with your fingers loosely stretched. Start breathing slowly and deeply. Imagine that your arms are growing loose, limp, and heavier with every breath you take.

Now imagine that your toes are loose pieces of rope dangling downward toward the ground. As you breathe in, feel and see your body filling up with

11

clean, clear, cool water. As you breathe out, see the tension in your body leaving with your breath. Feel your body getting heavier with each breath. Now let your legs go completely loose and limp; see every bit of tension drifting away; feel the pleasant sensation of relaxation spreading throughout your body.

CHAPTER 5
STRUCTURAL ALIGNMENTS

As we examine the qualities of each of the following exercises, I recommend that you spend at least 30-60 minutes a day for a full week or more on each individual quality until they become habits before you move on to the next exercise.

"Suspend" by the Top of Your Head

Begin by standing with your feet shoulder-width apart with your arms hanging at your sides. Let your whole body settle and relax in this position.

Next, imagine that the crown of your head is being pulled upward by wires. Your crown is located by tracing a line from the apex of your ear on each side of your head to the top of your head. (In acupuncture, this point is referred to as GV-20.) Where the two points meet at the center line is your crown.

Some of you may remember the Krazy Glue commercial showing a man hanging from a beam by his hard hat. Invest your mind in the image and recreate it mentally yourself. Feel the wires pulling up the top of your head while the rest of your body hangs free in space. You'll feel your neck extending in the way a turtle extends its neck. At the same time, you'll feel your body weight being pulled down by gravity.

Your chin should be tucked; that is, rotated slightly downward and inward until you feel a slight stretch in your neck. In doing this, you'll notice that the curvature of your neck will be reduced. Often people who do this exercise feel an immediate release of pressure in their shoulders and in their neck area.

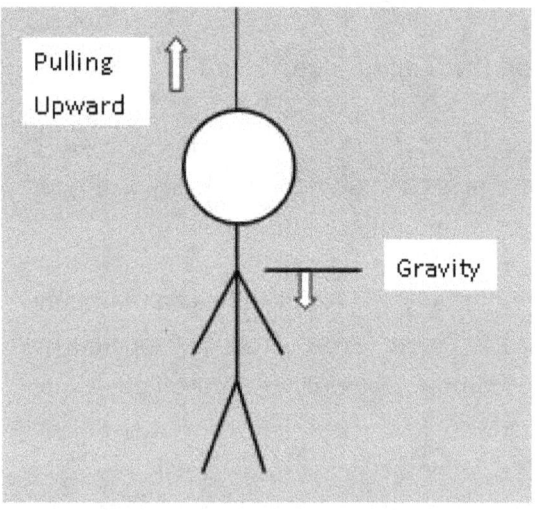

Feel your body hanging in space while gravity pulls your weight downward

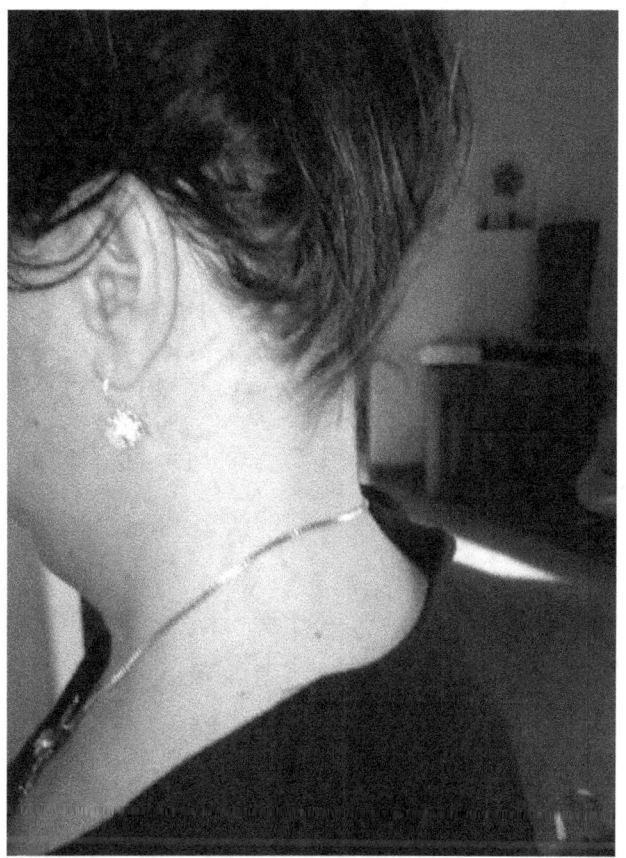

**Correct neck alignment resulting from suspension
exercise.**

Notice the straight neck line that "suspending"
yourself from the top of your head (via your
imagination) helps create. Extending your neck
helps relieve pressure on your cervical spine.
Frequently people suffer neck and shoulder pain as
a result of extending their jaw forward or from
continually looking downward at computer screens.
Both create compression of the cervical vertebrae.

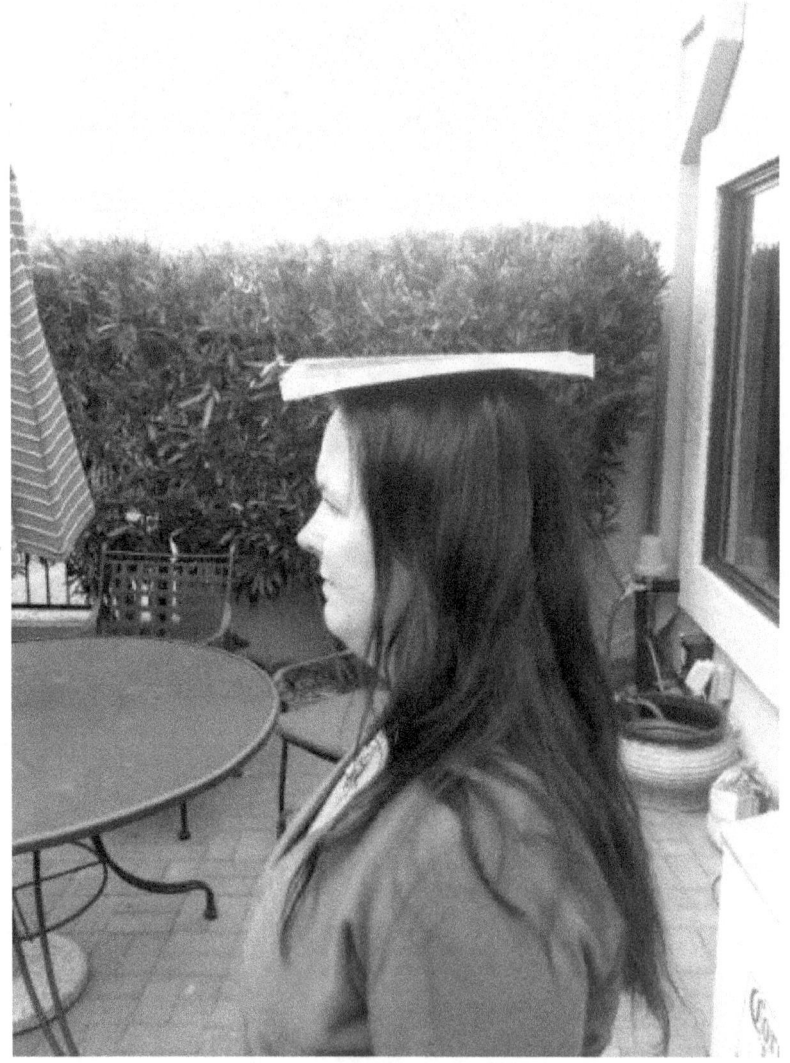

The balancing book exercise.

Another exercise that encourages good neck posture
is the book balancing exercise. This is a simple
exercise of balancing a book on your head as you
walk. By consistently practicing this exercise, you'll
develop a habit of good neck alignment in a

relatively short time. This exercise was commonly taught in finishing schools during the early part of the 20th century to help correct posture.

Again I emphasize that you should spend time practicing this exercise to get the full benefit of proper neck alignment. When you can easily balance a book on your head while stationary, add movement to your exercise by walking forward and backward, paying close attention to your alignment during the exercise.

Heavy Feet and Legs

Start this exercise with your legs a comfortable width apart. Allow your body to relax by visualization. Imagine that you can see into your body. Visualize that your body is a series of hollow tubes. Notice that the upper portion of your body, from the waist up, is separated from your hips and legs by a spigot of some sort which can be opened and closed at will.

As you look down your legs (using your imagination), you see they're completely hollow, all the way into your feet and toes. Now imagine that your upper body is full of sand. Mentally turn the spigot to your waist to allow the sand to start spilling into your feet.

See your feet expanding with the sand as they become heavier and heavier. Now notice that your feet are completely filled with sand and that more sand is beginning to fill your legs. You can see the shiny white grains of sand falling from your waist into your lower legs.

You now notice that the sand is falling faster and faster. Your thighs begin to feel like two large water balloons. As your thighs continue to fill with sand, you feel your legs growing heavier and heavier. You see the last few grains of sand fall from your waist down into your thighs. You feel the tremendous weight of the sand pulling your legs and feet down into the ground as if you're wearing concrete boots. As you look into your upper body and arms, you notice they're completely empty and feel incredibly light and free to move.

By doing this exercise on a regular basis, you'll notice that your range of motion will increase without stretching or pulling.

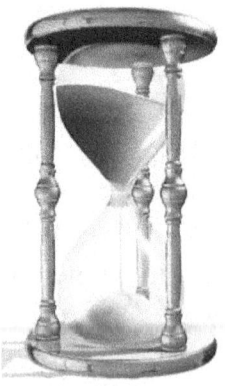

Allow all the weight in your upper body to drop completely into your legs.

Dragon Waist

Ever seen a reptile with a waist? This old Chinese idea tells us that our lumbar area should be straight.

So tuck your butt in—or, more precisely—roll your lumbar region downward and slightly inward until your lower back is straight.

You can practice this position while standing or sitting. Keep in mind it takes lots of **repetition** to retrain your body.

When you practice this sitting down, first tuck your butt in and then carefully sit down while maintaining the tucked position. Most people have the tendency to let their butt roll out behind them when they sit causing an outward curvature in the lumbar region. Train your low back to this new position slowly and gently. By working at it in this way you will make consistent progress.

You should experience a slight tightening sensation in your abdominal area which, if done correctly, will generate the sensation of heat during the exercise.

Practice for five to ten minutes while sitting, two or three times a day. As with the other concepts, practice this position until it becomes automatic and you no longer have to instruct your body to assume the position.

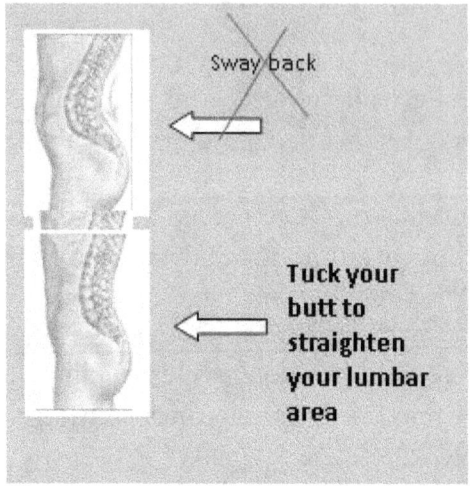

Using the concept of "dragon waist" allow your hips to tuck under your torso to straighten the lumbar region.

Monkey Back

When I mention having "a monkey back" I mean that your upper back area, from the bottom of your shoulder blades to the base of your neck, should be rounded until your scapula lies completely flat on your back.

One way to test for correct monkey back is to run your fingers over your scapula. If you can't grasp the scapular crests with your fingers, your position is correct.

The area between your shoulder blades extends as your upper back opens up. (Your back will appear much wider than before you started the exercise.) The loosening of your upper back allows your chest to become concave, forming a "pigeon chest".

You'll also notice that your shoulders 1will move
forward and your shoulder joints and arms will
move more freely. Notice the relaxed rounding of
your back and chest area.

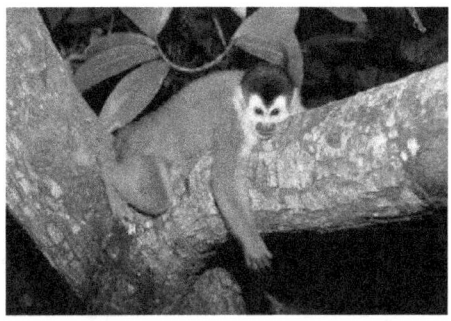

**A perfect example of "monkey back" and "pigeon
chest".**

Pigeon chest

This position gets its name from the concavity that
occurs when a bird beats it wings downward. The
principle of pigeon chest allows you to loosen the
pectoral and intercostal muscles that surround your
rib cage and lungs. This position helps straighten
your spine in the middle and upper area and relieves
the pressure on your shoulder joints.

To get a feel for pigeon chest, hollow your chest or
hold your hand against your chest to form a cavity.
You should notice as you do this that the shoulder
muscles across the top part of your back will loosen
and elongate, which allows your shoulder blades to
lay flat against the body. Breathe deeply as you do
this exercise and as you exhale see and feel the

tension leaving your body.

Another way to practice this position is to hug a good-sized tree. You'll notice the circular formation your upper body displays when you do this.

By continual practice of this exercise you can break up the tension that resides in and around the thoracic vertebrae.

As you get used to this position, you'll also notice that your shoulder joints will be looser and your arms will move more freely.

Keep in mind that all of these alignment qualities can be done while sitting, walking, or lying down. In fact, I encourage you to try all three positions!

CHAPTER 6
SUNG

Sung literally means "to relax and sink". *Sung* is a crucial concept in Tai Chi and can be only learned through practice.

To study this concept, stand with your feet shoulder-width apart, feet facing forward. If your feet are positioned correctly, it will appear as if you're slightly pigeon-toed (toes pointing slightly inward).

Allow your body to relax and let your arms hang to your sides. Maintain the idea of being suspended from the top of your head, as before. Now imagine that your feet are extremely heavy; imagine wearing concrete boots or standing in thick mud. Another effective image is to imagine roots extending from the bottom of your feet deep down into the ground.

Continue to feel the sensation that your feet are rooted deeply into the ground. Feel how cool and moist the soil is many inches below your feet. Feel the roots of your feet wrapping around rocks, penetrating deeper and deeper into the ground.

As you see and feel the roots going deeper, notice that your feet feel anchored to the earth. The sensation feels almost magnetic, as though your feet are held in place by magnets.

Notice that everything above your feet seems to move freely while your feet remain locked in place. This is the beginning of the concept of *sung*.

As you practice these images routinely, you should start to notice that you can drop your weight down into your legs and feet quickly.

After you get a feel for this exercise expand your sung by slowly walking around the room while maintain the sensation of your feet being locked to the floor. Use your focused attention with every step.

Practice sung every chance you get, waiting in line, at work, or at parties.

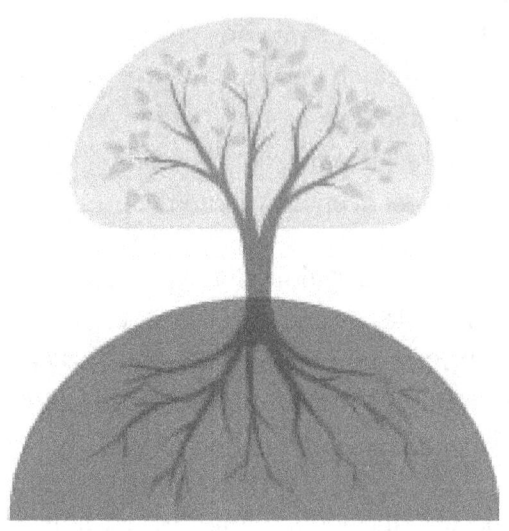

Sung exercise or rooting

By continuing to practice the suspension and foot exercises daily, after about seven days your body will embrace them automatically. Once you've developed this structural habit, you should feel your spine being stretched and elongated. As you do these exercises, you'll notice that your spine will feel looser and more agile. It isn't at all uncommon to hear people who have practiced this method for a while say that suddenly they feel taller and that their neck seems longer now.

You should also notice, after doing all these exercises for a period of time, that your feet will feel more rooted to the floor and that your *sung* has increased.

Now it's time to put all these ideas together into a standing position called Quiet Standing.

CHAPTER 7
QUIET STANDING

Quiet Standing is a form of standing meditation used to incorporate all of the principles you learned into a standing position to help quiet your mind. Quiet Standing is the beginning posture of the Yang Style form; it is often practiced as a solo Tai Chi exercise.

Stand with your heels together, toes facing outward at about a 15 degree angle (forming a V position). Make sure your feet are comfortable. Now apply all of the principles you've learned: top-of-head suspension, heavy feet, dragon waist, monkey back, and pigeon chest. Allow your arms to hang to your sides. Allow your body to sink and relax into the position. Let your knees bend slightly until they feel soft and springy. Close your eyes to limit distraction.

Start out standing in this position for 5 minutes a day; work up slowly to one hour a day. Allow your body to loosen to the point that you feel like you can almost fall forward. Approach the verge of falling; barely hold yourself in position. (Please Note: This position should be equally relaxed in all the compass positions—front to back and side to side.)

Allow your body to take on the quality of a sapling that bends easily at the top yet remains strongly rooted in the soil.

One of the best places to practice this exercise is outside. Find a secluded quiet area where you won't be disturbed and practice your Quiet Standing.

As your ability to relax improves, your awareness of your surroundings will also increase.

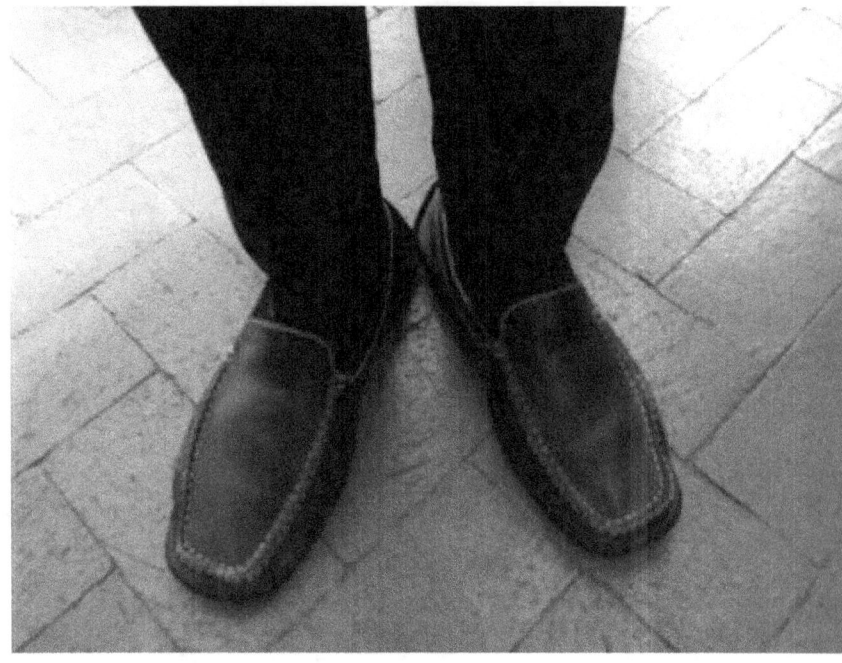

Quiet standing position.

Alternatively, stand with your feet shoulder-width apart, feet facing forward. Again relax and allow your arms to fall to your sides. Your fingers should be slightly opened and relaxed.

As you relax your upper back, you should feel a dry

sensation in your arm pit area. Let your weight completely sink into your feet. Let your body become completely loose and limp, to the point you almost feel as though you might topple over. Your body may start trembling or moving on its own. Allow it to do its thing. You may also notice the sensation of heat. These processes are all part of the effects of tension being released from your body. Realize that 70% of your body is made up of water and water moves freely in a container.

Quiet standing is a very old exercise and many Tai Chi masters have stated that quiet standing contains the very essence of Tai Chi. In fact many high level teachers do this one exercise exclusively as their primary Tai Chi practice.

I want to reemphasize the importance of keeping *your attention* focused while doing these exercises. Many people either neglect this essential point or are unsure what they should be doing mentally during standing.

Meditation is not a form of spacing out and letting your mind wander. Rather it is a form of focused **attention** on a given subject.

If you want to make progress and get the most out of your Quiet Standing pick out one aspect of the exercise to work on in a given session.

For instance one week you may choose to work on suspended head top and the next monkey back. Just put your attention on the exercise you want to develop and imagine it happening. Your mind will do the work for you.

Remember imagination always wins the day!

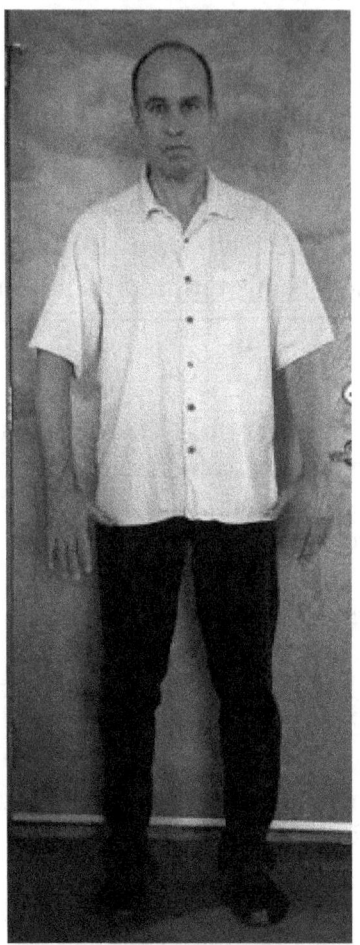

Quiet standing.

Check your body with a full length mirror to make sure your body is perfectly vertical, not leaning forward or backward, and that your spine is straight. Stand in either one of these positions for at least 5 minutes a day. Remember to completely allow your body weight to sink into your legs. Gradually increase your time up to 30 minutes a day and to notice positive changes in your body.

As you progress with aligning your posture to the tai chi principles, you may notice changes: more energy, more movement in your spine, a release of pressure on joints, your feet will feel heavy, and your body will feel light.

To get the maximum benefit from your Quiet Standing practice, learn belly breathing.

CHAPTER 8
BELLY BREATHING

Most people tend to breathe superficially (high up in the chest); they don't activate their diaphragm muscles.

In Tai Chi belly breathing, as we inhale we engage the diaphragm muscles by consciously expanding the abdomen outward. As we exhale, we consciously contract the diaphragm muscles inward.

As you practice this breathing, imagine seeing the air flowing into your belly and filling it up like a balloon. So, as you breathe in, fill the balloon and as your breathe out, deflate the balloon.

To enhance this exercise, apply your hand, palm down, to your navel area and see if you can get your hand to move. By continual practice you'll loosen your diaphragm muscles and begin to notice that your breathing is smoother and deeper. This exercise also massages your internal organs. After consistent conscious practice of this exercise for 7 days, your body will automatically do it without your help. When you're comfortable with belly breathing, apply it to your Quiet Standing routine.

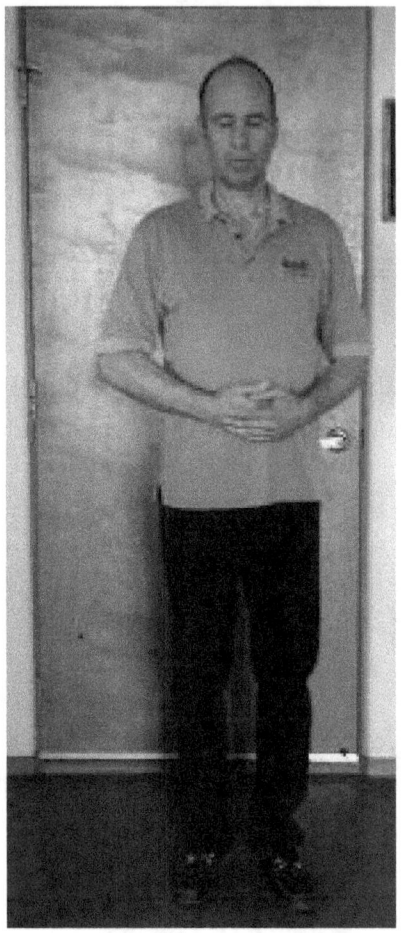

Belly Breathing Exercise

CHAPTER 9 TREE STANDING

Another, more advanced, standing position is known as tree
or pole standing. This exercise is done much like Quiet
Standing.

Make sure you have all the alignment qualities down before you work on tree standing.

Start this exercise by separating your legs shoulder-width apart, feet facing forward. Bring your arms up to shoulder position and make a circle as if you're hugging a tree. Allow your elbows to become extremely heavy and feel the weight of gravity pulling them downward.

Imagine a set of wires wrapped around your wrist and running to the ceiling. See and feel the wires holding your wrists, to the point that it feels like you're not even supporting your arms consciously.

Now allow your knees to bend and bring your body slightly forward on the ball of your feet. Activate your belly breathing. Stand in this position once a day for 5-10 minutes; work up to 1 hour. This exercise will build tremendous strength in your posture and will unlock your energy.

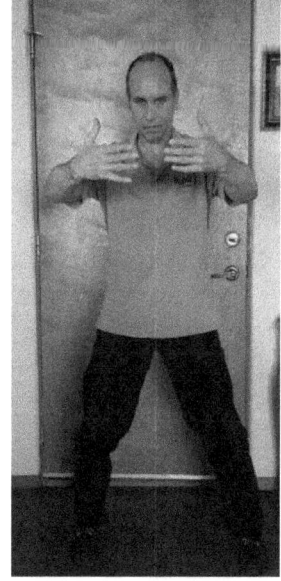

CONCLUSION

Your nervous system is a high-speed communication system that lives inside your body. Your nerves conduct electrical signals, called impulses, between your brain and body. Nerve impulses can be easily disrupted by spinal compression or restricted blood flow.

Compression is often due to the repetition of restrictive body positions caused by injury or mental tension. Body pain is one of the first signs of restricted blood flow and is often due to mental tension, trauma, malnutrition, and poor posture (to name a few factors). Long-term damage to nerves can result with effects ranging from reduced energy, to depression, to dizziness, and to shifts in overall health.

Building a strong, supple posture requires repetition. Remember: you are working with your mind and imagination and imagination always trumps willpower. **Your mind loves consistency. Do these exercises daily, going over one at a time. Read these chapters often. Relaxation puts you into a receptive state.**

Once you get the alignment qualities down, you can have fun developing your postural strength in other positions like the one shown below. As long as you're adhering to Tai Chi principles, you can practice your postures anywhere: riding the bus, in the swimming pool, in bed, lying down, sitting, even in an airplane. Get creative and realize there is no end to the possibilities.

ABOUT THE AUTHOR

Dr. David Money is a martial artist and licensed Doctor of Oriental Medicine in Santa Fe, New Mexico. He became actively interested in the healing arts in 1977 when he began studying Chinese martial arts under the guidance of an accomplished martial artist. After years of intensive study with several notable teachers and observing the outstanding effects that Tai Chi, herbs, and acupuncture produced in patients and students, he opened his clinic, Catalina Acupuncture, and started the Mind Form Technology Project which conducts ongoing research into how the mind influences the healing process.

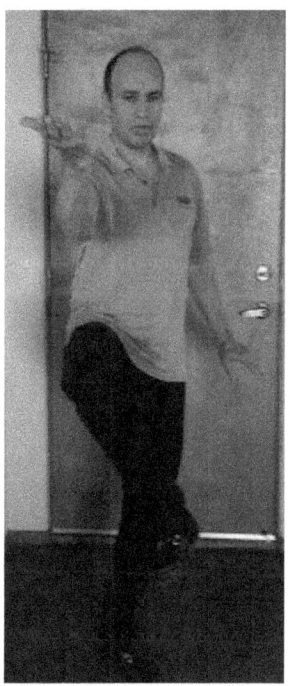

With a little imagination, you can practice Tai Chi-based relaxation 12 hours a day!

References

Cheng Tzu's Thirteen Treatises on T'ai Chi Chuan by Cheng Man Ch'Ing, Benjamin Pang Jeng Lo and Martin Inn, 1993.

Tao of Yiquan: The Method of Awareness in the Martial Arts by Jan Diepersloot, 2000.

Hole's Essentials of Human Anatomy & Physiology by David N. Shier, Jackie L. Butler and Ricki Lewis, 2006.

The Tao Teh King, Or The Tao And Its Characteristics. 1895.
by Lao-Tse
Translate by James Legge

Tao Te Ching by Lao Tsu. Sixth Century B.C
Translation by Gia-Fu Feng and Jane English. 1972.

The Essence of Tai Chi Chuan: The Literary Tradition. 1989.
Translation by Benjamin P. Lo Martin Inn), Susan Foe, Robert Amacker